Dr. Earl Mindell's

What You Should Know About Natural Health for Women

Dr. Earl Mindell's

What You Should Know About Natural Health for Women

Earl L. Mindell, R.Ph., Ph.D.

Keats Publishing, Inc. New Canaan, Connecticut

Dr. Earl Mindell's What You Should Know About Natural Health for Women is intended solely for informational and educational purposes, and not as medical advice. Please consult a medical or health professional if you have questions about your health.

Library of Congress Cataloging-in-Publication Data

Mindell, Earl.
  [What you should know about natural health for women]
  Dr. Earl Mindell's what you should know about natural health for women / by Earl Mindell.
    p.   cm.
  Includes bibliographial references and index.
  ISBN 0-87983-754-3
  1. Gynecology—Popular works. 2. Naturopathy.
3. Generative organs. Female—Diseases—Alternative treatment. 4. Herbs—Therapeutic use. 5. Menopause—Hormone therapy. I. Title.
RG121.M665 1996
618.1—dc20   96-19146
                                                CIP

Printed in the United States of America

Keats Publishing, Inc.
27 Pine Street (Box 876)
New Canaan, Connecticut 06840-0876

98 97 96   6 5 4 3 2 1

CONTENTS

ACKNOWLEDGMENTS

This book would not have been possible without the pioneering work of Dr. John R. Lee, M.D., and his book *What Your Doctor May Not Tell You About Menopause: The Breakthrough Book on Natural Progesterone,* the most complete information available on the use of natural hormones.

Introduction

Because I am a pharmacist as well as a nutritionist and herbalist, I have a unique point of view on natural health and alternative medicine. I have first-hand knowledge of how drugs work in the body, how they are prescribed, and why doctors prescribe the drugs they do. I am not going to do too much "doctor bashing" in this book, and I acknowledge that by and large, medical doctors are well-meaning, if misguided in their approach to health care. But women's health in North America is an area of the health care system that is fraught with danger for many women.

It is an embarrassing misconception that America has the world's greatest health care system, and nowhere does this apply more than in women's health. Here are a few telling facts and numbers:

Our infant death rate is still worse than that of 22 other countries.

Our rate of death from heart disease is the highest in the world, and women make up a large part of that statistic.

U.S. doctors perform some 500,000 unnecessary hysterectomies each year, condemning those women to the prison of hormone replacement therapy for life. (You can imagine what a big business half a million hysterectomies every year is for the makers of Premarin and Provera!)

According to the Centers for Disease Control and Prevention, U.S. doctors performed 349,000 unnecessary cesarean deliveries in 1991, at a cost to the nation of $1 billion, and at a cost to mothers of severe pain and scarring, the risk of major surgery, a higher rate of infections, and longer hospital stays. In the world, only Brazil and Puerto Rico have higher rates!

Heart disease is the number one cause of death in women over the age of 70, but this wasn't known until recently because only men were invited to participate in heart disease studies and women weren't being diagnosed and treated for heart disease. (Women are too complicated—they have menstrual cycles, they get pregnant and they go through menopause. Women of child-bearing age aren't asked to be in many studies because most of the studies are designed to test drugs which may carry the risk of pregnancy complications and birth defects.)

THE "PILL FOR EVERY ILL" MINDSET

The information you are exposed to in the media and from your doctor tends to be shamefully awash in misleading drug company advertising and marketing fictions that can be harmful to your health, and even increase your risk of death. I'm going to tell you about some of these misconceptions and dangers in this book, and give you some safe, effective, natural solutions for health problems experienced by many women.

I want you to understand, for the sake of your health, that nearly all doctors are unduly influenced by drug companies from the time they're in medical school until the day they retire. Even medical school curriculums are extremely biased toward the disease/drug approach to health care. In medical school doctors are first taught anatomy and physiology, then they are taught how to diagnose disease, then they are taught what drug to prescribe to treat a disease. Their approach to medicine and healing is very limited and narrow and with a primary focus on symptoms.

Also starting in medical school, doctors are courted, cajoled and bribed with expensive meals, gifts, equipment, vacations and free drugs by the pharmaceutical company sales reps. Doctors in practice may be given the "incentive" of a free vacation or expensive gift if they sell a certain amount of a drug.

Once a doctor is in practice, most of his or her information about drugs is going to come from drug company sales reps—the average doctor just doesn't have time to keep up with the latest medical journals. This is why doctors practice medicine under seemingly incredible misconceptions and fallacies that a simple glance at a biochemistry textbook could correct. For example, there's a common misconception that menopause is caused by a drop in estrogen, and that estrogen is an anti-aging hormone. The truth is that menopause is much more complicated than being an "estrogen deficiency disease" and in excess estrogen is the opposite of an anti-aging drug. But more about that later.

To make matters worse, insurance companies have gotten into the business of practicing medicine, and may refuse to cover a patient's treatment if the doctor doesn't prescribe the drug approved by the insurance company for treating that disease. This problem is even more exaggerated in an HMO, which may itself dictate the standards of care. If M.D.s don't follow those so-called "standards" they run the risk of losing their job, their medical license or their hospital privileges. For a doctor fresh out of medical school, half a million dollars in debt, and probably with a family to support, these are potent incentives to toe the line and forget the facts.

There is very little genuine care and concern for your health and well-being among the drug companies. The closest you'll come to concern from the typical health care organization is a desire not to be involved in a lawsuit.

With this knowledge, it's easy to understand how a doctor may be unduly influenced to prescribe drugs. In the past century, our medical system has created a very powerful M.D. mindset that says there's a pill for every ill. But the first vow of a new doctor is to "do no harm," and buying into drug company hype and handing out pills for every ill is a sure way to inflict damage on patients. My fervent hope is that as patients become increasingly disenchanted with a medical system that's not working they'll turn to alternative sources of healing and medicine, and the M.D.s will be forced to change their ways or become extinct.

Important health matters such as the causes and prevention of illness, the role of nutrition in illness, and the role of the mind and emotions in illness, are either completely ignored in medical school, or given a few token hours. Ironically, it's difficult or impossible to help people stay healthy without taking the above factors into account. The good news is, there's change in the wind. Some insurance companies and HMOs are coming to the realization that they could save literally millions of dollars a year in health care costs by simply paying attention to preventive care practices such as educating patients about nutrition and a healthy lifestyle. Nearly all of our common chronic diseases such as heart disease, diabetes and arthritis are completely preventable.

THE PSYCHOLOGY OF GOING TO THE DOCTOR

Something else you should be aware of is the psychology of going to the doctor. All too often, the real reason people go to the doctor is because they're having problems in their personal lives, and they don't know where else to turn. They go to the doctor with some minor complaint, hoping in some vague way that the doctor will fix their problem, or at least give them some comfort and attention. But going to the doctor is likely to make you sick! Patients don't like to walk away from a doctor's office without a prescription, and doctors like to please their patients, and that can be the start of a long battle with ill health. You'll take the prescription for say, an allergy drug, an antacid, an H2 blocker, some antibiotics, a pain killer, a sleeping pill, and your symptoms go away for awhile.

But pretty soon you're noticing other symptoms, which are caused by the first prescription, so you go to the doctor again, and get another prescription, which causes a new round of side effects. Pretty soon you're spending hundreds of dollars a month on drugs and you feel terrible, and it never occurs to you that the symptoms could be caused by all the drugs. And all you went in for in the first place was a chronically stuffy nose, or heartburn, symptoms that might have easily been handled by kicking the cat off the bed or giving up on those greasy French fries!

My advice to you is to avoid going to the doctor as much as possible. All illness is caused by an imbalance of some kind in the body. Most of those imbalances can be brought back into balance with lifestyle changes and nutritional healing. We are far more intelligent and knowledgeable about our bodies than we give ourselves credit for. Developing an awareness of what you're doing to create that ache or pain is a key to good health.

Unless you are acutely ill, or have acutely serious symptoms, before calling for a doctor's appointment, ask yourself: am I doing everything I can to keep my life balanced and whole? Am I eating well, getting some exercise, taking some vitamins, and spending time with loved ones or helping others? Am I living a life of moderation and balance? Am I drinking too much alcohol or too many sodas? Could I give up that third and fourth cup of coffee? Am I eating plenty of fresh vegetables? Am I avoiding pesticides indoors and outdoors? Could I give up that doughnut I have for breakfast? Do I need to spend more time taking care of myself and less time worrying about the health of my loved ones? Could I reduce the stress in my life? Would I feel better if I had a heart-to-heart talk with my husband? If you have moderate symptoms that have been bothering you for awhile, you can track down the cause yourself, nearly all the time.

If you're unable to track down the cause of your ill health, or you're looking for a tune-up for optimal health, I suggest you see a naturopathic doctor, a chiropractor (many of them use nutrition and herbs for healing and balancing the body), or an M.D. specializing in alternative medicine. They are more likely to work with you in a balanced way that addresses more than symptoms and drugs. I will certainly go to an M.D. if I have a broken bone, and I'll certainly use antibiotics if I have pneumonia, but these are very much the exceptions. Most of us are only suffering from the consequences of our bad habits, and that can be fixed!

CHAPTER 1

Hormones and How They Affect You

Your body's biochemistry is a beautiful, complex and intricately balanced system that is largely still way beyond the comprehension of science and medicine. One of the most important and finely tuned systems in your body, which profoundly affects every other system in your body, is the steroid hormones. Other hormones in the body include insulin and growth hormone (and even vitamin D is considered a hormone), but in this book we'll stick to the steroid hormones.

The steroid hormones include pregnenolone, progesterone, DHEA (dehydroepiandrosterone), the estrogens, the androgens, the cortisols and testosterone. You probably recognize these as the hormones secreted by your ovaries and your adrenal glands.

The building block for all of these hormones is cholesterol, which is in turn made from the breakdown products of foods you eat. The steroid hormones regulate and play a part in a seemingly endless list of functions in the body, including our sex characteristics, our sex drive, thyroid metabolism, insulin regulation, blood pressure, behavior and moods, inflammation, allergies and on and on.

These hormones work together, and when one is out of balance, the others tend to follow, so you can imagine how important it is to help your body maintain hormone balance. Let's take a brief look at some of the hormones.

ESTROGEN: THE HORMONE OF FEMININITY AND CELL DIVISION

Estrogen is actually the name of a class of hormones. Some of its better-known members are estradiol, estriol and estrone. To confuse matters, the drug companies refer to their weird not-found-in-nature estrogen-like drugs as estrogens. But don't be fooled. Premarin, for example, is made from a plant-derived human estrogen and a pregnant mare-derived estrogen. This is called a conjugated estrogen, but it certainly doesn't resemble anything found in the human body!

When girls reach puberty and begin to experience bodily changes such as growing breasts, underarm hair and pubic hair, as well as the unseen changes of development of the uterus, vagina and fallopian tubes, estrogen is the hormone driving these changes. It is also responsible for a woman's curves, those extra deposits of fat that aren't particularly popular in our culture at this time. (At one time they were considered the height of beauty and femininity.) When a young woman's estrogen levels, along with the levels of other hormones, rise high enough, she will begin ovulating and having menstrual periods.

Like her other hormones, a woman's estrogen will ebb and flow during the course of her menstrual cycle. Estrogen is highest at the beginning and middle of the cycle, when it is stimulating the uterine tissue to grow, providing a rich, blood-filled womb for embryo growth. This property of stimulating cell growth is both what makes estrogen a feminine hormone, and what makes it dangerous when it is found in the body in excess, or unbalanced by progesterone. Estrogen doesn't just stimulate cell growth in the uterus; it can also stimulate the growth of cells in breast tissue, ovarian tissue and cervical tissue.

Estrogen also causes the body to retain water. This accounts for its ability, when it is the dominant hormone, to cause weight gain, bloating, irritability, headaches, and other brain symptoms such as foggy thinking, memory loss and depression.

ESTROGEN DOMINANCE

Dr. John R. Lee, the leading authority on the use of natural progesterone to balance hormones, has coined the term "estrogen dominance" to describe what happens when a woman has an imbalance of hormones characterized by estrogen unbalanced by the hormone progesterone. Even if a woman's estrogen levels have dropped, say at menopause, if her progesterone levels have dropped even further, her hormones will be unbalanced and she will suffer from estrogen dominance. In other words, it's not an estrogen excess per se that causes estrogen dominance, it's too much estrogen relative to not enough progesterone.

Both women who have suffered from PMS and women who have suffered from menopausal symptoms will recognize the hallmark symptoms of estrogen dominance: weight gain, bloating, mood swings, irritability, oversensitivity, tender breasts, headaches, fatigue, depression, hypoglycemia, clumsiness, uterine fibroids, endometriosis, and fibrocystic breasts, just to name the more common symptoms.

Because progesterone is supposed to be the dominant hormone during the premenstrual phase of a woman's cycle, for years PMS was blamed on progesterone. Ironically it is precisely a *deficiency* of progesterone that is causing the problem, at a time in the cycle when it was supposed to be dominant.

Dr. Lee believes that many illnesses that afflict women in the U.S. are caused by estrogen dominance, including uterine fibroids, breast, ovarian and uterine cancer, fibrocystic breasts, hypoglycemia, low thyroid, gallbladder disease, autoimmune diseases such as lupus, and miscarriages.

With progesterone playing such an important role in hormone balance, let's examine it more closely.

I'll talk more about estrogen, menopause and hormone replacement therapy in the section on menopause.

PROGESTERONE: THE HORMONE OF PREGNANCY AND BALANCE

Progesterone is the building block of all the other steroid hormones. In contrast, estrogen is an end-point hormone, meaning no other hormones are made from it. Progesterone's primary role as a hormone precursor means that a deficiency of progesterone can result in a deficiency or imbalance of other steroid hormones, throwing the entire body out of balance. This is why symptoms of PMS and menopause can be so severe for some women.

In the female body, progesterone is made in the ovaries, the adrenal glands, the placenta during pregnancy, and even, some researchers speculate, in the brain. The ovaries produce the vast majority of a woman's progesterone, on a monthly cycle. But the production of progesterone is dependent upon ovulation. Without ovulation, there is no ovarian progesterone. How does that work?

Each month a follicle, which is a sac inside the ovary containing an egg, migrates outside the ovary and ruptures, releasing the egg. The egg then begins its journey down the fallopian tube to the uterus, while the ruptured sac, now called the *corpus luteum,* produces progesterone. If for some reason ovulation doesn't happen that month, there is no progesterone made by the corpus luteum, which is a setup for estrogen dominance.

Rising progesterone levels at mid-cycle have the effect of maturing the cells of the uterine lining that estrogen has stimulated to grow, preparing them either for an embryo or to be shed in menstruation. When pregnancy doesn't occur, the brain sends out signals to the ovaries, and both progesterone and estrogen levels fall, creating the end of a menstrual cycle with the shedding of the uterine lining.

Dr. Lee theorizes that the ability of progesterone to mature cells may partly account for its potential to prevent and even reverse reproductive cancers in women, and, I might add, in men. And remember, I am not talking about the synthetic progestins here, which seem to stimulate cancerous growth.

WHY AREN'T WOMEN OVULATING?

There are many reasons women don't ovulate. Perhaps the most common is simply stress. Our bodies are intimately and intricately connected to the brain, and the brain's response to stress is to signal the body not to reproduce. Another common reason for non-ovulatory cycles, called *anovulatory* cycles, is strenuous exercise. Many women athletes don't ovulate, and some don't even menstruate. Is it possible not to ovulate and still have a menstrual period? Absolutely! That just means there is enough estrogen to stimulate the uterine lining to build and then shed its blood-rich tissue. A lack of menstruation means there isn't enough estrogen in the body to stimulate tissue growth in the uterus, so there's nothing to shed at the end of the cycle.

The consequences of anovulatory cycles are serious: all of the estrogen dominance symptoms can come into play, including uterine fibroids and fibrocystic breasts, as well as endometriosis. Weight gain, fatigue, depression, sleep disturbances, and foggy thinking can dog the heels of a woman who's not ovulating. And she may not even be aware of it because she's continuing to have menstrual periods.

Progesterone is also the primary hormone of pregnancy. After about the third month, the placenta begins producing progesterone, and by the third trimester the placenta is producing 300-400 mg of progesterone every day! This is a whopping dose for a hormone!

Progesterone also plays a large part in sex drive, or libido, which is logical, since it is the hormone present in the greatest amount at ovulation, when a woman is fertile.

THE THREAT OF XENOESTROGENS

Let's digress from the subject of progesterone for a moment to talk about *xenoestrogens*. According to Dr. Lee, one cause of anovulatory cycles is "follicle burnout" caused by xenoestrogens, which are environmental estrogens that come from pesticides, herbicides, fungicides, some types of soap, air pollution, plastics, and from the meat of animals that are fattened for slaughter with estrogen-like drugs, an almost universal practice in the United States. These xenoestrogens are not identical to estrogen, but are enough alike so that they behave somewhat like estrogen in the body. They are usually very potent, and are especially dangerous to a growing fetus because they can cause reproductive abnormalities that show up later in life.

Remember, in addition to creating female characteristics, one of estrogen's primary jobs in the body is to stimulate cell growth. Xenoestrogens may very well be a cause of the rising rates of reproductive organ cancer (for both women and men), including breast cancer, testicular cancer, ovarian cancer and cervical cancer, as well as the rapidly dropping sperm count in men, and the epidemic of infertility among couples in their thirties.

I strongly encourage you to avoid xenoestrogens as much as possible. You can do that by:

√ Eating organic fruits and vegetables whenever possible;

√ Never spraying your garden or lawn with pesticides, herbicides or fungicides (there are plenty of effective ways to control pests without pesticides);

√ Never spraying or "bombing" your home with insecticides;

√ Minimizing your consumption of meat unless you know it's hormone-free;

√ Using environmentally friendly soaps that do not contain nonylphenols, a type of surfactant;

√ Not cooking in plastic, which sheds when heated.

WHY ISN'T NATURAL PROGESTERONE USED IN HORMONE REPLACEMENT THERAPY?

Many doctors would answer the above question by saying, "Of course progesterone is used in hormone replacement therapy! What do you think Provera is? What do you think the progestins are?"

And herein lies a misconception that has caused harm to millions of women. The progestins such as Provera (medroxyprogesterone acetate) are most emphatically not the same as progesterone. They are synthetic versions of progesterone, molecules not found in nature, and the body does not respond to them in the same way it does to the natural progesterone found in your body. They're close, but close doesn't count in hormones. The molecular difference between testosterone and estrogen is less radical than the difference between progesterone and the progestins, and yet the difference between testosterone and estrogen is the difference between a man and a woman!

If your doctor argues with you on this, point out the following: remember that the placenta produces 300-400 mg of progesterone during the last few months of pregnancy, so we know it's the ultimately safe hormone to have in the body during pregnancy. But the progestins can cause birth defects with a fraction of those amounts! I'd hardly call that the same hormone! The progestins also cause many other side effects, including partial loss of vision, breast cancer in test dogs, an increased risk of strokes, fluid retention, migraine headaches, asthma, cardiac irregularities, depression and a whole list of other side effects caused by combining it with the synthetic estrogens.

Natural progesterone, on the other hand, has never been shown to have any side effects except sleepiness at very high doses.

If you're not a reader of my newsletter, you may be asking why the drug companies would produce a drug with that many side effects when the real thing is easily available and cheaper, with no known side effects, and even more appalling, why the FDA ever approved it? The answer is money. Natural progesterone can't be patented because it's a natural substance, and therefore the drug companies can't charge outrageous prices for it. So they create a synthetic, patenable drug, pretend it's the same thing, and drop millions and millions of advertising and marketing dollars into perpetuating the illusion that the two are the same. Even most doctors believe it!

Now you see why I'm telling you over and over again

that neither the drug companies nor the FDA are looking out for your best interests. You must take the initiative to educate yourself and protect your own health.

WHERE DOES NATURAL PROGESTERONE COME FROM?

There is an enormous amount of confusion about exactly what a natural progesterone is. My definition is the same as Dr. Lee's: that is, to be called progesterone, it must be the same molecule as the progesterone made in a woman's body.

But the progesterone used for natural hormone replacement doesn't come from people, or from animals; it comes from either diosgenin, extracted from a very specific type of wild yam *(Dioscorea spp.)* that grows in Mexico, from a substance extracted from soybeans called stigmasterol, or from cholesterol derived from wool fat.

In the laboratory, diosgenin, stigmasterol and cholesterol can relatively easily and cheaply be converted to the exact molecular structure of all of the human steroid hormones, including estrogen, testosterone, progesterone and the cortisones. And in fact, this is where nearly all pharmaceutical hormones originate.

IS WILD YAM EXTRACT THE SAME AS PROGESTERONE?

Some companies are trying to sell diosgenin, which they label "wild yam extract" as a medicine or supplement, claiming that the body will then convert it into hormones as needed. This is a very neat and logical-sounding theory, and I wish it were true, but unfortunately there no evidence that this is what happens. There are piles of papers proving this can be done in the laboratory, but nothing showing that's the way it happens in the human body. I keep hearing promises that "research is under way that is going to prove this," but it never surfaces.

Diosgenin or wild yam has been used by herbalists to relieve menstrual cramps, abdominal pain, and it has been shown in studies to lower cholesterol a little bit, so it may very well be a useful medicinal plant. I just want you to avoid the notion that it will have the same effect as progesterone cream, or that by taking it you are taking progesterone, or any of the other steroid hormones, for that matter. In addition, wild yam is used in Mexico as a fish poison so I would avoid taking it in high doses if you should decide to try it.

Unfortunately the consequences of this type of "theoretical marketing" can be tragic. I recently got a call from the owner of a health food store, telling me that a woman was in his store in a wheelchair, demanding to know why the progesterone she was taking hadn't helped her osteoporosis. She had taken a bone density measurement, faithfully used progesterone cream as instructed, and here she was six months later with a hip fracture caused by a minor fall, and lower bone density than when she started.

My friend was puzzled, having seen many good results with progesterone and osteoporosis. I told him to ask her what brand of progesterone cream she was using. Well, it turns out she wasn't using a progesterone cream at all, she was using a diosgenin cream labeled as "wild yam extract" and advertised as giving all the benefits of progesterone. Please don't make this mistake—the consequences are too serious. And by the way, to confuse matters even further, real progesterone cream is often labeled "wild yam extract," so the best thing to do is know your sources. I will give you a list of reliable sources of natural progesterone cream at the end of the book.

HORMONES AND MENOPAUSE

I'll go into more detail on using natural hormones at menopause in the section on menopause. But right now I want you to know that estrogen is not the hormone most women need to be taking for menopausal symptoms. Estrogen will do most women more harm than good, making them feel great for a few months, and then dropping them into a kind of permanent postmenopausal PMS.

Estrogen levels only drop 40-60 percent at menopause, which is just enough to stop the menstrual cycle. But progesterone levels may drop to near zero in some women. In a healthy woman, hormone levels will fall off very gradually, over time, with a gradual lessening of menstrual cycles, and with very little in the way of menopausal symptoms.

Menopause is relatively uneventful in most Third World countries, and in Japan there's not even a name for hot flashes! According to Dr. Lee, this is because the high-stress, high-calorie and low-exercise lifestyle of most American women creates higher-than-normal hormone levels, which drop more abruptly at menopause, creating the unpleasant symptoms of hot flashes and night sweats, along with all the estrogen dominance symptoms.

In the menopause chapter of this book I'll talk in more detail about a lifestyle for a healthy menopause.

THE MALE HORMONES

Although testosterone is the hormone that confers "maleness," women also have some testosterone in small amounts. Testosterone, along with progesterone, plays an important role in sex drive. It also builds bone, helps define muscle, and speeds up metabolism.

DHEA (dehydroepiandrosterone) is an important hormone mainly made by the adrenals, which also tends to be an androgen, or male hormone. It is clear that some men can benefit from DHEA supplementation, as high as 150 mg a day, as they age, but less clear with women, as very little research has been done with women. However, there is some indication that older women may benefit from 20 mg a day of DHEA. Please don't take high doses of DHEA. The research we do have indicates it may increase insulin resistance and the risk of heart disease in women at high doses. And again, please do not take diosgenin or "wild yam extract," thinking you are getting DHEA. As far as we know that doesn't happen reliably.

CHAPTER 2

Naturally Healthy Breasts

Women's breasts are very sensitive to hormones, and particularly to estrogen and progesterone. Women who experience breast tenderness premenstrually will attest to this.

Virtually every risk for breast cancer is associated with excessive estrogen in some way. This makes sense, because estrogen stimulates tissue growth, and particularly tissue in the breasts and reproductive organs.

According to the American Cancer Society, more cancers are detected by women examining themselves than by mammogram. This is a simple, effective routine that should be done by every women, every month, for her entire life. It's best to do a breast exam just after a menstrual period, so that premenstrual breast lumps can be distinguished from lumps that are independent of monthly cycles.

FIBROCYSTIC BREASTS

Some estimates are that 60 percent of women in their premenopausal years experience fibrocystic breast changes. The symptoms include lumps and tenderness. Some women have many lumps, some women only have one. Fibrocystic breasts generally worsen premenstrually. When menopause begins, fibrocystic breasts end, in most women.

The breasts are composed of fatty tissue interwoven with ducts and glands for milk. Breast ducts

19

and glands are the parts of the breast influenced by hormones, particularly estrogen, which stimulates duct growth and branching. If they are overstimulated, they can become swollen and blocked, leading to the formation of cysts. Fibrocystic breasts are probably caused by estrogen dominance, and can nearly always be relieved with the use of some progesterone cream.

Assuming that if you have fibrocystic or tender breasts you're premenopausal, you can use the recommended dose of progesterone cream (usually ¼ to ½ tsp) daily, from day 12 of your cycle (day 1 is the first day of menstruation) to two days before your period is due, usually 26 to 28 days for most women. **Do not** use progesterone cream if you are trying to become pregnant, because starting the cream before you ovulate can block ovulation, and stopping it at day 26 or 28 brings on menstruation because it is an abrupt drop in hormones that triggers menstruation.

If you are under the age of 35, I recommend that you try dietary and lifestyle changes, and some herbs, before resorting to progesterone. (Women over 35 should try these remedies first too, but they are more likely to have a progesterone deficiency leading to estrogen dominance.)

MOVE THAT LYMPH SYSTEM!

Exercise is one of the best things you can do to relieve tender or fibrocystic breasts. Moving your body moves your lymphatic system, which is composed of millions of tiny channels, glands and ducts that transport toxins out of the body. One of the primary lymph gland sites is under the armpit, near the breasts.

The lymphatic system moves when you do. Stretching is one of the best types of exercise you can do for your lymph system. Many yoga, tai chi and chi gong movements are specifically designed to move the lymphatic system.

DIET FOR HEALTHY BREASTS

There are a few basic dietary changes that have helped many women reduce or eliminate fibrocystic breasts. Perhaps the most important is cutting out coffee. For some reason coffee in particular seems to aggravate fibrocystic breasts, probably because it's so hard on the liver. Many women have eliminated their problem simply by eliminating coffee.

It may seem contradictory to tell you to drink plenty of water when water retention can aggravate breast tenderness, but water is your body's favorite cleanser. Drink at least 6–8 glasses of clean water daily when you are premenstrual.

Another important step is eliminating hydrogenated oils such as are found in margarine, and nearly all processed baked goods and chips. These synthetic oils block important biochemical pathways of essential fatty acids, promoting inflammation. It's also important to avoid processed, unsaturated vegetable oils, which are usually rancid by the time they get onto your dinner table. Stick to the monounsaturated oils such as olive oil and canola oil, and small amounts of saturated oils such as butter and coconut oil. Yes, contrary to popular opinion, saturated fats are perfectly fine as long as you eat them in moderation. They shouldn't comprise more than 10 percent of your fat and oil consumption. I would much rather have you eat butter than margarine or other hydrogenated oils!

Meat is a good food to go easy on when you are premenstrual. It takes a lot of energy to digest meat, and you'll avoid those estrogen-like drugs that are

used to fatten cattle, as well as the pesticides (xenoestrogens) that become concentrated in fatty tissues.

Eating fish a couple of times a week, as well as
plenty of nuts, fresh fruits and vegetables, and whole
grains, will give you the essential fatty acids you need.
You can take an essential fatty acid supplement too.
These are usually derived from evening primrose oil
or borage oil, and fish oils.

HERBS FOR FIBROCYSTIC BREASTS

Although fibrocystic breasts are most likely caused by
hormonal imbalances, once you have them you're
dealing with inflammation and tissues that have, in
effect, become clogged or toxic. Some of the herbs
I'm going to recommend are for hormonal balance,
and some are for detoxification. The liver is the organ
most responsible for excreting excess estrogen, so it's
very important to specifically support your liver. Since
the liver has to expend a lot of energy to get rid of
excess fat, you can also support your liver by strictly
avoiding fried foods, and keeping your fat intake
moderate.

Check your health food store for formulas and teas
made from these herbs. They can be very effective in
relieving symptoms and helping your body restore itself to normalcy.

All of these herbs can be taken as a tincture, tea or
capsule, following the directions on the container.

Black Cohosh (Cimicifuga racemosa)

This is one of the ultimate women's herbs, used extensively by the American Indians for menstrually related
problems. It contains phytoestrogens (plant estrogens
which occupy estrogen receptor sites, lessening the effect of the body's estrogen), and many other nutrients

which strengthen and balance the female reproductive system. Black cohosh nourishes the adrenals and kidneys, improves circulation, is calming, helps relieve the swelling caused by water retention, and improves digestion.

This is not an herb to use if there is a possibility you are or may become pregnant.

Dandelion (Taraxacum off.)

Sore, tender breasts can often be caused or aggravated by water retention. In this case a diuretic, which helps the body eliminate excess water, can be very helpful. Dandelion is a wonderful medicinal herb that is a gentle diuretic and contains helpful minerals, including potassium. It is also high in lecithin, a substance that supports liver function, your most important route of detoxification.

Vitex/Chasteberry (Vitex agnus castus)

Traditionally, chasteberry was very popular in Europe as a woman's remedy for regulating the reproductive system, treating PMS, and unpleasant symptoms associated with menopause such as hot flashes.

Research has revealed the presence of a volatile oil in chasteberry which tends to balance the production of women's hormones. This oil is believed to contain a progesterone-like substance, which could explain the herb's therapeutic effect in relation to PMS symptoms such as anxiety, nervous tension, insomnia, and mood changes, as well as tender breasts and cramping. Chasteberry has also been used to treat irregular menstruation, heavy bleeding and fibroid cysts. Vitex needs to be taken regularly over a period of at least a month or two to have its effect.

Yellow Dock (Rumex crispus) and Milk Thistle (Silybum)

These are both wonderful herbs for supporting and tonifying the liver. When you support your liver, your body will rid itself of toxins more quickly.

Sage (Salvia officinalis)

Named from the Latin for "to save," sage has been associated for centuries with longevity. It has a long-standing reputation as an aid for painful periods and tender breasts, and it will aid in the digestion of fat. Other cooking herbs such as rosemary and thyme also have a beneficial effect on fat digestion.

Besides its powerful oils, sage contains estrogenic compounds (which can soften the effect of excessive estrogen by taking up estrogen receptor sites on cells). It also contains antibacterial agents and antioxidants.

Sage should only be taken as remedy for a week or two at a time, since it has another substance, thujone, which can have potentially toxic effects. Please don't mistake "garden sage" for desert sage (Artemesia tridentata).

White Willow Bark (salix alba)

For pain relief, white willow bark tea, capsules or tincture can provide the same analgesic effect as aspirin without the stomach distress caused by aspirin. Willows have been tapped since antiquity for pain relief and reduction of fever. Ancient manuscripts of Egypt, Greece, and Assyria refer to willow bark, and even Hippocrates recommended willow to counter pain.

SUPPLEMENTS FOR HEALTHY BREASTS

It is important to maintain a good daily vitamin regimen (see my book in this series, *What You Should Know*

About Creating Your Personal Vitamin Plan), for optimal nutritional support. In addition, the following supplements will help prevent tender and fibrocystic breasts.

Vitamin B6 will help balance hormones because it is an important part of the body's process of transforming one hormone into another. Without adequate B6 your body may be unable to make the hormones it needs to keep everything in balance. Vitamin B6 will also help relieve water retention. Take 50 mg two times a day between meals.

Calcium and Magnesium are important for maintaining proper fluid balance in the cells and for muscle relaxation. Be sure you're getting 1,200 mg of calcium and 400–500 mg of magnesium daily.

CHAPTER 3

Naturally Healthy Monthly Cycles

A woman's monthly cycles are perfectly designed by nature to prepare the body for impregnation. We call them monthly cycles, but they more accurately represent the lunar cycle of the moon.

At the beginning of a cycle, prior to ovulation, the brain is releasing hormones that instruct the uterus to build a thick, blood-rich lining stimulated by estrogen, which will act as a temporary incubator for an embryo should the monthly egg be released and fertilized. By the end of the third trimester the placenta will be fully surrounding and protecting the fetus, and starting to produce progesterone in copious amounts.

Around the middle of the cycle, called the luteal phase, the brain again signals the ovaries, this time to release a follicle, which is a sac inside the ovary containing an egg. One follicle makes it to the surface of the ovary and releases an egg. While the egg is making its way down the fallopian tube where it may meet up with sperm, the empty follicle sac, now called the corpus luteum, is releasing progesterone. At this point in the cycle, both progesterone and estrogen levels are fairly high.

When impregnation doesn't happen, progesterone levels and estrogen levels begin to drop, falling abruptly at the end of the cycle, around day 26, and stimulating the uterine muscles to contract and release their bloody lining.

What I've just outlined above is a very simplified

version of a woman's monthly cycle, and while the body is adept at adjusting for all kinds of variations, from diet to stress, there are many ways this cycle can be thrown out of balance.

MENSTRUAL CRAMPS

It is likely that nearly all women have experienced menstrual cramps, what doctors call dysmenorrhea, at some time in their life, but for some women, an estimated 10 percent, their monthly cycles are a source of pain and misery that will cause them to miss work and school. Up until recently, the medical mindset toward menstrual cramps was that they were psychologically caused and women should just endure them or take a pain killer. Of course this is not true. Cramps can be made worse by stress, but they are caused by very real biochemical imbalances in the body.

Menstrual cramps may have more than one cause, but the primary one is an excess of "bad" prostaglandins called PGF2, which are normally released to stimulate gentle muscle contractions of the uterus, allowing the shedding of the uterine lining, or endometrium. In excess, the muscle contractions become cramps.

An excess of "bad" prostaglandins is primarily caused by doing things that block the "good" prostaglandin pathways. The prostaglandin pathways are largely regulated by our intake of essential fatty acids (EFAs). Eating hydrogenated oils (found in margarine and most baked goods and chips) and rancid oils can block the EFAs, starting a chain reaction down the bad pathways. Many women can avoid cramps simply by avoiding hydrogenated oils and limiting their oils to olive oil, canola oil and butter.

A diet high in refined carbohydrates and sugar will also drive oils down the bad pathways. Viral illnesses and excessive adrenal hormones secreted in response to stress can also create more bad prostaglandins and a deficiency of good ones. This is why we can accurately say that stress does contribute to menstrual cramps.

Some doctors will prescribe birth control pills to relieve menstrual cramping. If they help, this is an indication that the cramps may be caused by estrogen dominance—an imbalance of estrogen caused by a progesterone deficiency. In this case it would be far safer to use the natural hormones found in progesterone cream. To use progesterone cream, follow the directions given in the chapter on naturally healthy breasts. However, if you are under the age of 35, it is far preferable to try the lifestyle and dietary changes recommended first. You might use progesterone cream for a few months while you are getting your system back in balance, but always try the simplest solutions first.

THE CRAMP-FREE DIET

To balance your prostaglandins you need a balanced intake of EFAs. This means eating fish two or three times a week, and including a variety of nuts (except peanuts), seeds, whole grains and fresh vegetables in your diet. You also need to minimize your intake of coffee, diary products, red meat and alcohol, all of which will stimulate the bad prostaglandins.

Taking an EFA supplement can significantly help prevent menstrual cramps. These will come in the form of GLA and EPA supplements. The EPA usually comes from fish, and the GLA from borage oil. You only need 1–2 mg of GLA and 50–100 mg of EPA oils. Take them starting at least a week before your period is due.

Pain killers such as aspirin and ibuprofen help relieve the symptoms of menstrual cramps by blocking both prostaglandin pathways. This will provide symptomatic relief for some women, but suppressing the good prostaglandins has the effect of suppressing the immune system. These types of drugs are also very hard on the stomach. I suggest you work to correct the underlying cause of your cramps and bring your body back into balance.

I recommend the book *Women's Bodies, Women's Wisdom* by Christiane Northrup, M.D. (Bantam, 1994) for an in-depth look at how the emotional and stress-related causes of menstrual cramps can be healed.

If you use tampons, be sure they aren't the cause of your cramps. Try a couple of cycles without them and see if that helps. Gas and constipation can aggravate cramps, so when you are premenstrual, try to avoid foods that cause those symptoms.

HERBS FOR MENSTRUAL CRAMPS

Herbs can be very useful for gently and safely relieving the pain and muscle spasms of menstrual cramps. Please do not use them if you are trying to get pregnant, as some of them can encourage menstruation. Some women can experience cramping as an early sign of pregnancy.

As always, use herbs in moderation, follow the directions on the container, and be cautious about mixing them with other drugs. Herbs are generally much safer than prescription drugs, but it always pays to be cautious. All of the herbs listed here can be taken as teas, tinctures or in capsule form. You can also check your health food store for formulas made specifically for menstrual cramps that contain some or all of these plants.

In this section, and later in the book, you will notice that some information is repeated. This is because certain herbs and nutrients operate on several conditions, and the full information should be available in each place where it will be called for, even if it also appears elsewhere.

Anise (Pimpinella anisum)

This common plant is mainly an antispasmodic, used for relieving the muscle spasms associated with menstrual cramps. You can chew on anise seeds, drink it as a tea, or take it in capsules.

Cramp Bark (Viburnum opulus)

This aptly named bush will help relieve cramps anywhere in the body. It relaxes muscles and nerves.

Chamomile (Matricaria chamomilia)

Chamomile makes a mild, relaxing and soothing tea that can help promote menstruation when it is delayed.

Dong Quai (Angelica sinensis)

This is one of the most-used Chinese herbs for balancing women's hormones. It works specifically on the uterine muscles, and appears to contract or relax them, as needed, to bring balance. These types of herbs are known as "adaptogens," because they tend to bring the body into balance. Contrary to popular opinion, dong quai does not contain estrogen-like substances, or have an estrogenic effect on the body. It has a mild sedative effect, a mild diuretic effect, and enhances liver function.

Sage (Salvia officinalis)

Sage has a long-standing reputation as an aid for painful periods. Besides its powerful oils, sage contains estrogenic compounds (which can soften the effect of excessive estrogen by taking up estrogen receptor sites on cells). It also contains antibacterial agents and antioxidants.

Sage should only be taken as remedy for a week or two at a time, since it has another substance, thujone, which can have potentially toxic effects. Please don't mistake "garden sage" for desert sage *(Artemesia tridentata)*.

White Willow Bark (salix alba)

For pain relief, white willow bark tea, capsules or tincture can provide the same analgesic effect as aspirin without the stomach distress caused by aspirin. Willows have been used since antiquity for pain relief. Ancient manuscripts of Egypt, Greece, and Assyria refer to willow bark, and even Hippocrates recommended willow to counter pain.

SUPPLEMENTS FOR MENSTRUAL CRAMPS

As mentioned above, taking an essential fatty acid (EFA) supplement can significantly help relieve menstrual cramps. It is important to maintain a good daily vitamin regimen (see my book in this series, *What You Should Know About Creating Your Personal Vitamin Plan*), for optimal nutritional support. In addition, the following supplements will help prevent menstrual cramps.

Vitamin B6 will help balance hormones because it is an important part of the body's process of transforming one hormone into another. Without adequate B6 your body may be unable to make the hormones it needs to keep everything in balance. Vitamin B6 will also help relieve water retention. Take 50 mg two times a day between meals.

Calcium and Magnesium are important for maintaining proper fluid balance in the cells and for muscle relaxation. Magnesium is one of the most effective remedies for muscle spasms. Be sure you're getting 1,200 mg of calcium and 400–500 mg of magnesium daily. You can double your magnesium intake the week before your period. Be sure to take it in a buffered form or it can cause diarrhea.

Vitamin E has been shown to help prevent and relieve menstrual cramps. You should be taking 400 mg daily as part of your daily vitamin regimen. You can add another 400 IU for the week before your period.

Bioflavonoids can help reduce the inflammation associated with some menstrual cramping. There are many bioflavonoid formulas available. Some of my favorite bioflavonoids are quercetin, grapeseed extract and hesperidin.

CHAPTER 4

Natural Solutions for PMS

PMS, or premenstrual syndrome, has achieved wide recognition in the past few decades. Like menstrual cramps, PMS was first thought to be a product of a woman's unbalanced psyche. Now we know it can be caused by a complex interplay of factors that include genetics, nutrition, hormones and stress.

It is estimated that 50 percent of all women experience mild PMS, but my guess would be that nearly all women have experienced some form of PMS between the time menstruation begins and menopause. An estimated 30 percent of women experience moderate PMS symptoms, and some five percent experience symptoms that are severe enough to interfere with their daily lives.

PMS symptoms occur a week or ten days before menstruation begins and go away shortly after. They include a lot of "mental/emotional" symptoms such as depression, weepiness, anxiety, irritability, foggy thinking, memory loss, confusion, inability to focus, and anger. Other symptoms include clumsiness, dizziness, fatigue, headaches, muscle aches and pains, water retention and the resulting weight gain, nausea, low back pain, acne, breast tenderness, and food cravings, particularly for chocolate, sugar, and refined carbohydrates such as cakes and cookies.

Women who suffer from PMS dread those times of the month, and so do their family and friends. If you look at Dr. John Lee's list of estrogen dominance symptoms, and look at a list of PMS symptoms, you'll find they are very similar. Katharina Dalton, a British M.D., pioneered the use of progesterone for PMS decades ago. She had great success in relieving symptoms, but the vaginal or rectal suppositories she used to deliver the hormone were not popular.

Meanwhile, back in the U.S. many doctors were blaming progesterone for causing PMS, because that was the dominant hormone present at the end of the menstrual cycle. Somehow it never occurred to them that a progesterone *deficiency* could be causing the symptoms!

Many women can relieve their PMS symptoms by using some natural progesterone cream, but it should not be treated like a magic bullet. Severe PMS symptoms are the body's way of letting you know that something is very much out of balance, and if you fail to address those imbalances, they will reappear somewhere else in the body.

There are a variety of factors that can contribute to PMS. A thyroid deficiency can imitate many PMS symptoms, including headaches, fatigue and mental fogginess. Women who have allergies, who abuse alcohol, or have chronic gastrointestinal problems are more prone to suffer from PMS. Lack of exercise will contribute to PMS. I'm sure that pervasive petrochemical pollution and the resulting prevalence of xenoestrogens (potent environmental estrogens) are also contributing to PMS.

REDUCE STRESS LEVELS

Stress can certainly push a woman who is on the edge, over the edge into PMS. Chronic stress stimulates the release of adrenal hormones that in excess can throw the rest of the body's hormones out of balance and block the good prostaglandin pathways (see the chap-

ter on naturally healthy monthly cycles for more information on prostaglandins). Women whose PMS
symptoms include cramping and abdominal pain are
likely to be especially susceptible to stress.

To uncover the sources of your stress, it can help
to talk to a sympathetic friend or relative, or even a
therapist, who is willing to listen and help you sort
things out. Good nutrition, exercise, plenty of sleep
and a life that is balanced with work and play, will go
a long way towards reducing stress. Meditation or the
Eastern disciplines of yoga, tai chi or chi gong can
also greatly help relieve stress. Again, I recommend
Dr. Christiane Northrup's book, *Women's Bodies, Wom-
en's Wisdom* (Bantam 1994) for good advice on han-
dling stress.

Women who suffer from cramps as part of their
PMS symptoms should read the chapter on a naturally
healthy monthly cycle, paying particular attention to
the section on essential fatty acids and prostaglandins.

DIET FOR A PMS-FREE MONTH

Poor nutrition is a primary factor in aggravating PMS.
The PMS-free diet is similar to the diet for healthy
breasts and a healthy menstrual cycle. These few basic
dietary changes have helped many women reduce or
eliminate their PMS symptoms.

The most important step you can take is eliminating
hydrogenated oils such as are found in margarine and
nearly all processed baked goods and chips. These synthetic oils block important biochemical pathways of
essential fatty acids, promoting inflammation. It's also
important to avoid processed vegetable oils, which are
usually rancid by the time they get onto your dinner
table. Stick to the monounsaturated oils such as olive
oil and canola oil, and small amounts of saturated oils
such as butter and coconut oil. Coconut oil is perfectly

good for you when eaten in moderation. It is high in medium-chain triglycerides, beneficial oils that can help balance prostaglandins.

The next most important step you can take is to eliminate the very foods many women crave, namely sugary, highly refined carbohydrate foods such as cakes, cookies and candy. This will only aggravate the insulin and blood sugar imbalances caused by excess estrogen. Taking the supplements listed below will greatly help reduce sugar cravings. Try eating some fresh fruit, or raw carrot sticks when a sugar craving comes on.

Meat is a good food to go easy on when you are premenstrual. It takes a lot of energy to digest meat, and you'll avoid those estrogen-like drugs that are used to fatten cattle, as well as the pesticides (xenoestrogens) that concentrate in fatty tissue. Protein in general seems to aggravate PMS symptoms. It may help to eat primarily vegetarian foods and fish when you are premenstrual.

Eating fish a couple of times a week, as well as plenty of fresh fruits and vegetables and whole grains, will give you the nutrients and fiber you need. Fiber is an important part of a PMS-free diet, because it helps the body eliminate toxins, including excessive estrogen.

It's very important to drink plenty of water to assist your body in detoxifying itself and staying hydrated. Dehydration in itself can cause cramping, headaches and irritability. Drink at least 6–8 glasses of clean water daily when you are premenstrual.

HERBS FOR A PMS-FREE MONTH

Herbs can play a major role in preventing and treating PMS symptoms. Please do not use them if you are trying to get pregnant, as some of them can encourage menstruation. Some women can experience cramping as an early sign of pregnancy.

As always, use herbs in moderation, follow the directions on the container, and be cautious about mixing them with other drugs. Herbs are generally much safer than prescription drugs, but it always pays to be cautious. All of the herbs listed here can be taken as teas, tinctures or in capsule form. You can also check your health food store for formulas made specifically for PMS that contain some or all of these plants.

Black Cohosh (Cimicifuga racemosa)

This is one of the ultimate women's herbs, used extensively by the American Indians for menstrually related problems. It contains phytoestrogens (plant estrogens which occupy estrogen receptor sites, lessening the effect of the body's estrogen), and many other nutrients which strengthen and balance the female reproductive system. Black cohosh nourishes the adrenals and kidneys, improves circulation, is calming, helps relieve the swelling caused by water retention, and improves digestion.

This is not an herb to use if there is a possibility you are or may become pregnant.

Dandelion (Taraxacum off.)

PMS can often be aggravated by water retention. In this case a diuretic, which helps the body eliminate excess water, can be very helpful. Dandelion is a wonderful medicinal herb that is a gentle diuretic and contains helpful minerals, including potassium. It is also high in lecithin, a substance that supports liver function, your most important route of detoxification.

Dong Quai (Angelica sinensis)

This is one of the most-used Chinese herbs for balancing women's hormones. It works specifically on the uterine muscles, and appears to contract or relax them, as needed to bring balance. These types of herbs are known as "adaptogens," because they tend to bring the body into balance. Contrary to popular opinion, dong quai does not contain estrogen-like substances, or have an estrogenic effect on the body. It has a mild sedative effect, a mild diuretic effect, and enhances liver function.

Ginger (Zingiber spp.)

Ginger is one of the most versatile plants on earth, being widely used both as a medicinal plant and as a spice. Its major action is to stop cramping, especially in the digestive system and in the uterus.

Ginger is best known for its effectiveness in relieving indigestion and most types of nausea. Researchers believe it is ginger's mild suppressing effect on the central nervous system that prevents nausea, and this would also account for its ability to relieve PMS symptoms. Ginger can relieve some migraine headaches, which often occur premenstrually in women. Ginger also contains antioxidants, anti-inflammatory and anti-bacterial substances. It has been used to help regulate heartbeat and like aspirin, but without its side effects, it reduces the tendency of blood to clump, thus reducing the risk of heart attacks and strokes. As well as using fresh ginger root in food or to make a tea, you can also take it in a powdered form in capsules.

Vitex/Chasteberry (Vitex agnus castus)

Traditionally, chasteberry was very popular in Europe as a woman's remedy for regulating the reproductive system, treating PMS and unpleasant side effects associated with menopause such as hot flashes.

Research has revealed the presence of a volatile oil in chasteberry which tends to balance the production of women's hormones. This oil is believed to contain a progesterone-like substance, which could explain the herb's therapeutic effect in relation to PMS symptoms such as anxiety, nervous tension, insomnia, and mood changes, as well as tender breasts and cramping. Chasteberry has also been used to treat irregular menstruation, heavy bleeding and fibroid cysts. Vitex needs to be taken regularly over a period of at least a month or two to have its effect.

Yellow Dock (Rumex crispus) *and Milk Thistle* (Silybum)

These are both wonderful herbs for supporting and tonifying the liver, an important part of maintaining hormone balance, and preventing PMS. When you support your liver, your body will rid itself of toxins more quickly.

SUPPLEMENTS FOR A PMS-FREE MONTH

It is important to maintain a good daily vitamin regimen (see my book in this series, *What You Should Know About Creating Your Personal Vitamin Plan*), for optimal nutritional support. In addition, the following supplements will help prevent PMS symptoms

Essential Fatty Acids (EFA) can significantly help relieve PMS. Take a supplement with a two-to-one ratio of EPA oils to GLA oils. Flax seed oil can be taken for a week or so premenstrually to relieve symptoms, but I don't recommend it be taken every day long-term because it can suppress both good and bad prostaglandin pathways. Also always make sure that flax seed oil comes in a light-proof container, is refrigerated and dated, and don't use the same bottle for more than two weeks. Flax seed oil is one of the most unstable of all the unsaturated oils, and if it becomes rancid it will certainly do you more harm than good. To avoid the issue of rancidity, you can also buy the seeds and grind them just before you eat them.

Vitamin B6 will help balance hormones because it is an important part of the body's process of transforming one hormone into another. Without adequate B6 your body may be unable to make the hormones it needs to keep everything in balance. Vitamin B6 will also help relieve water retention. Take 50 mg two times a day between meals.

B-Complex vitamins can help with the mental/emotional symptoms of PMS. Take a B-50 complex the week before your period, in addition to your regular vitamins.

Calcium and Magnesium are important for maintaining proper fluid balance in the cells and for muscle relaxation. Magnesium is one of the most effective remedies for muscle spasms. Be sure you're getting 1,200 mg of calcium and 400–500 mg of magnesium daily. You can double your magnesium intake the week before your period. Be sure to take it in a buffered form or it can cause diarrhea.

Vitamin E has been shown to help PMS symptoms to some degree. You should be taking 400 IU daily as part of your daily vitamin regimen. You can add another 400 IU for the week before your period.

Bioflavonoids can help reduce the inflammation associated with some menstrual cramping. There are many bioflavonoid formulas available. Some of my favorite bioflavonoids are quercetin, grapeseed extract and hesperidin.

The Minerals copper, zinc, manganese, selenium and chromium should either be present in your multivitamin or taken as an additional supplement premenstrually. Chromium can help reduce sugar cravings. For those symptoms, take 200 mcg twice daily for the premenstrual week.

CHAPTER 5

A Naturally Healthy Urinary Tract

Urinary tract infections (UTIs) are one of the most common and painful infections that can plague women. Chronic UTIs are poorly handled by mainstream medicine. Most women get at least one UTI in their life, and it is estimated that as many as 20 percent of all women have a bout with chronic UTI.

A UTI can be caused by trouble in the kidneys, the bladder, or the urethra, the tube leading from the bladder through which urine is excreted. Most often the symptoms are caused by a bacterial infection in the urethra or bladder.

One of the first symptoms of a UTI can be a burning or cramping sensation in the lower abdomen or behind the pelvic bone. Other symptoms of a UTI are a burning pain on urination; urgency, or the feeling of a strong need to urinate frequently but only a small amount of urine is voided; and foul-smelling urine or blood and/or pus in the urine.

Symptoms such as vomiting, chills and low back pain may be a sign that the kidneys are involved. It is important to see a doctor if you have blood in your urine, vomiting, a high fever or chills.

The vast majority of UTIs are caused by bacteria that find their way up the urethra from the genital area, or a bladder infection, but this is only part of the story. In order for an infection to take hold, the urinary tract has to be out of balance.

One of the primary functions of the kidneys and

bladder is to eliminate bacteria from the body, so usually bacteria are washed out of the urethra when you urinate. In fact, urine itself will usually kill bacteria. A bladder infection usually involves some type of blockage or pooling of urine in the bladder. Thus it's clear that an imbalance must be present to create a UTI.

One such imbalance may be in the pH of the urine, or the acid/alkaline balance. Stress, poor diet and some medications, such as antibiotics, can throw off the pH of the urinary tract, creating a susceptibility to infection.

Too much protein is one of the biggest dietary offenders when it comes to UTIs. A high-protein diet produces an acidic condition in the body, which creates a high stress load on the kidneys. If the kidneys can't keep up, a UTI often results.

Sugar will also aggravate a UTI, so it's important to avoid sweets while you're healing an infection or if you're susceptible to chronic UTIs.

Pregnancy, diabetes, and a sudden increase in sexual activity can also trigger UTIs. Other contributing factors can be chronic dehydration; resisting the urge to urinate and delaying urination; diaphragms used for birth control; a yeast infection; and tight pants or sports such as horseback riding and bicycling, which may force bacteria up the urethra, irritate the urethra or block the flow of urine. It is also important to urinate soon after having sexual intercourse.

If your immune system is compromised by stress, poor nutrition, alcohol or drug abuse, excessive caffeine, and excessive sugar, it makes it much easier for a UTI find a hold in your body.

Some UTIs occur primarily in menopausal women. They are caused not by a bacterial infection, but by an estrogen deficiency that thins the tissue of the vagina and the urethra, and shrinks the genitalia. The thinning of tissue can cause easy bruising and tissue damage, creating the symptoms typical of a UTI. These types of infection can often be cured with a *natural* estrogen cream applied topically in the genital area.

Mainstream medicine tends to treat urinary tract infections with antibiotics, but in chronic cases with underlying imbalances, antibiotics only cause rebound infections and compromise the immune system as well as upsetting the digestive system. Antibiotics also encourage yeast infections, which can precipitate a UTI! Please don't resort to antibiotics unless the kidneys are involved, or the infection is serious.

REMEDIES FOR URINARY TRACT INFECTIONS

Your best treatment for a UTI is prevention, but if you get one, here are some safe, natural remedies you can try. Be sure to see a health-care professional if the symptoms are severe for more than a few days, if there is blood in your urine, or if you have a high fever, chills and pain in your kidneys or lower back.

One of the simplest and most important remedies is to drink plenty of clean water, up to 6–8 glasses a day. This may seem like the last thing you'd want to do when it hurts to urinate, but you need the cleansing action of water.

DIURETICS

Diuretics help encourage the flow of fluids through the kidneys, which cleanses the urinary tract. Diuretics should be used in moderation, since you also don't want to stress the urinary tract.

Bearberry (Uva ursi) is an honored old folk remedy for UTIs. It acts as a diuretic, antibacterial agent, and astringent. A tea is the most recommended way to take it, but tinctures and capsules are also available. Do not take more than the recommended dose of bearberry, as it can be toxic at high doses.

Parsley *(Petroselinum sativum)* is a diuretic and contains nourishing chlorophyll and minerals that are healing to the urinary tract. It also happens to be good for digestion and is a wonderful breath freshener. Do not drink parsley tea if you are pregnant or trying to become pregnant.

TO FIGHT INFECTION

Echinacea *(Echinacea angustifolia)* and **goldenseal** *(Hydrastis canadensis)* are powerful immunostimulants. Goldenseal is soothing to mucous membranes, and has antibacterial properties, so it is well worth trying in place of antibiotics if the infection is not serious.

Garlic *(Allium sativum)* is a potent antibacterial agent, especially against one of the most common UTI invaders, E. coli. Put raw garlic in your salad, use it in cooking, or if you don't like the odor, take the odorless capsules.

CRANBERRY JUICE

For decades the medical profession pooh-poohed the use of cranberry juice for fighting UTIs, but women never stopped using it, because it's such an effective remedy. Finally some studies were done showing that indeed, cranberry juice was effective in clearing up UTIs. The original theory was that cranberry juice acidified the urine, but scientists have since discovered that a substance in the cranberry prevents bacteria from clinging to the wall of the urethra, allowing them to be washed out during urination. Please don't buy cranberry juice heavily sweetened with sugars, including corn syrup or fructose, which will negate any good the cranberry is doing. Either mix it with the smallest possible amount of a sweeter juice, such as grape juice, or water it down enough so that you can drink it unsweetened. Drink at least two 8 oz glasses a day.

WARM BATHS AND COMPRESSES

A warm bath with aromatic oils or soothing minerals can work wonders to speed the healing process of a urinary tract infection. A hot water bottle or warm compress on the lower abdomen can also help relieve pain and soothe inflammation.

CHAPTER 6

A Naturally Healthy Premenopause

Many women today are suffering from what Dr. John Lee has coined "premenopause syndrome," caused by anovulatory (not ovulating) menstrual cycles in which no progesterone is made, creating a relative excess of estrogen and estrogen dominance (see the chapter on hormones for details). Anovulatory cycles may begin as early as a woman's early thirties, and can be a setup for years of seemingly undiagnosable symptoms.

A woman who is not ovulating can still be menstruating—she is still producing enough estrogen to cause the buildup of tissue in the uterus—but if she doesn't ovulate she won't be producing any progesterone.

Premenopause syndrome is particularly apt to occur in highly stressed women who are trying to maintain a career, a family and a marriage.

The symptoms of premenopause syndrome include weight gain, bloating, mood swings, cold hands and feet, irritability, unstable blood sugar, fatigue, and depression. Other symptoms are infertility, endometriosis, fibrocystic breasts and uterine fibroids. Premenopause syndrome is also a setup for osteoporosis, as the lack of progesterone, which stimulates bone growth, will result in loss of bone and decreased bone density. (The fact that osteoporosis begins at least a decade short of menopause is well documented.)

If premenopause symptoms are being caused by anovulatory cycles, then the straightforward solution is to supplement the body with natural progesterone in

49

the form of a cream. Because progesterone is fat-soluble, it is easily absorbed through the skin. The cream can be rubbed anywhere on the body, but areas where the skin is thin, such as the palms, inner arms, sides of the torso and upper inner thighs are probably best.

A progesterone cream delivers a fairly reliable dose. Oral progesterone is more problematic because most of it is promptly excreted by the liver before having any effect on the body. Therefore, to get a proper dose of 30–40 mg of progesterone daily, you have to take 100 to 200 mg of oral progesterone, in hopes that the liver will miss a small percentage of it. However, depending on diet, liver function, the toxin load on the liver and many other factors, the dose you actually get is unpredictable, and it is very easy to get too much progesterone, resulting in sleepiness. In addition, oral progesterone puts the liver to a lot of unnecessary work.

The progesterone cream should be used from day 12 to day 26 or 28 of the menstrual cycle (the first day of menstruation is day 1). When you stop using it, menstruation should begin within 48 hours. Please do not use progesterone cream without professional guidance if you are trying to get pregnant, as progesterone can influence ovulation, and the abrupt cessation of daily progesterone cream usually brings on menstruation.

Please follow the dietary and lifestyle advice in the chapters on naturally healthy breasts and natural healthy monthly cycles, for premenopause syndrome. The use of progesterone cream is addressing a symptom underlying a deeper problem that is blocking ovulation. Premenopause syndrome is a signal from the body that it is out of balance, and you need to address that imbalance on many levels.

For a detailed explanation of pre-menopause syndrome and other women's hormone balance issues, as well as detailed descriptions of how to use natural progesterone, I highly recommend the book, *What Your Doctor May Not Tell You About Menopause: The Breakthrough Book on Natural Progesterone,* by John R. Lee, M.D. (Warner Books, 1996).

HERBS FOR PREMENOPAUSE

Black Cohosh (Cimicifuga racemosa)

This is one of the ultimate women's herbs, used extensively by the American Indians for menstrually related problems. It contains phytoestrogens (plant estrogens which occupy estrogen receptor sites, lessening the effect of the body's estrogen), and many other nutrients which strengthen and balance the female reproductive system. Black cohosh nourishes the adrenals and kidneys, improves circulation, is calming, helps relieve the swelling caused by water retention, and improves digestion.

This is not an herb to use if there is a possibility you are or may become pregnant.

Dong Quai (Angelica sinensis)

This is one of the most-used Chinese herbs for balancing women's hormones. It works specifically on the uterine muscles, and appears to contract or relax them, as needed to bring balance. These types of herbs are known as "adaptogens," because they tend to bring the body into balance. Contrary to popular opinion, dong quai does not contain estrogen-like substances, or have an estrogenic effect on the body. It has a mild sedative effect, a mild diuretic effect, and enhances liver function.

Vitex/Chasteberry (Vitex agnus castus)

Traditionally, chasteberry was very popular in Europe as a woman's remedy for regulating the reproductive system, treating PMS and unpleasant side effects associated with menopause such as hot flashes.

Research has revealed the presence of a volatile oil in chasteberry which tends to balance the production of women's hormones. This oil is believed to contain a progesterone-like substance, which could explain the herb's therapeutic effect in relation to premenopause' symptoms. Chasteberry has also been used to treat irregular menstruation, heavy bleeding and fibroid cysts. Vitex needs to be taken regularly over a period of at least a month or two to have its effect.

Yellow Dock (Rumex crispus) *and Milk Thistle* (Silybum)

These are both wonderful herbs for supporting and tonifying the liver. When you support your liver, your body will rid itself of toxins more quickly.

SUPPLEMENTS FOR A NATURALLY HEALTHY PREMENOPAUSE

Essential Fatty Acids (EFA) can significantly help relieve premenopause symptoms. Take a supplement with a two-to-one ratio of EPA oils to GLA oils.

Vitamin B6 will help balance hormones because it is an important part of the body's process of transforming one hormone into another. Without adequate B6 your body may be unable to make the hormones it needs to keep everything in balance. Vitamin B6 will also help relieve water retention. Take 50 mg two times a day between meals.

B-Complex vitamins can help balance the mental/emotional symptoms of premenopause syndrome.

Take a B-50 complex, in addition to your regular vitamins.

Calcium and Magnesium are important for maintaining proper fluid balance in the cells and for muscle relaxation and for fatigue and weakness. Magnesium is one of the most effective remedies for muscle spasms. Be sure you're getting 1,200 mg of calcium and 400–500 mg of magnesium daily. You can double your magnesium intake the week before your period. Be sure to take it in a buffered form or it can cause diarrhea.

Vitamin E has been shown to help balance women's hormones to some degree. You should be taking 400 IU daily as part of your daily vitamin regimen, and you can add 400 IU when you have symptoms.

Bioflavonoids can help reduce the inflammation and relieve fatigue and weakness. There are many bioflavonoid formulas available. Some of my favorite bioflavonoids are quercetin, grapeseed extract and hesperidin.

The Minerals copper, zinc, manganese, selenium and chromium should either be present in your multivitamin or taken as an additional supplement premenstrually. Chromium can help reduce sugar cravings. For those symptoms, take 200 mcg twice daily for the premenstrual week.

CHAPTER 7

Naturally Healthy Menopause

Nothing gets commercialized faster or cashed in on faster in medicine than women's health problems. Pregnancy has been treated like a disease for nearly a century, and as a result the U.S. has one of the highest infant mortality rates in the industrialized world. Nearly half a million unnecessary hysterectomies are performed every year in the United States, condemning those women to a lifetime on hormone replacement therapy; a steady source of cash flow for drug companies and doctors, but a source of side effects and greater susceptibility to disease for the women.

Menopause is no exception. Since the 1960s the drug companies have been trying to convince doctors and women that menopause is, as Dr. John Lee has coined it, "an estrogen deficiency disease" that needs to be treated with synthetic, not-found-in-nature hormones.

Menopausal women are at higher risk of heart disease and osteoporosis, but I promise you, estrogen is not the solution! After an initial period of feeling better, estrogen and the synthetic progestins cause most women to feel as if they have permanent PMS! The not-found-in-nature synthetic hormones prescribed by most doctors do vastly more harm than good, and their ability to protect against heart disease and osteoporosis is grossly exaggerated by drug companies.

The problems associated with menopause are also grossly exaggerated by the drug companies and the media. In truth, it is women who have had a hysterectomy (instant menopause) who have the most problems. The vast majority of other women pass through menopause relatively uneventfully.

THE REAL STORY ON ESTROGEN

Estrogen has been touted by the drug companies and the media as an elixir of youth, but in fact, estrogen is more like the grim reaper. Progesterone levels actually drop much more dramatically at menopause than estrogen levels do, and this accounts for more of the menopausal symptoms than a drop in estrogen does.

Most articles on hormone replacement therapy do not distinguish between estrogen therapy alone, and estrogen combined with the synthetic progestins. Most of the beneficial effects attributed to estrogen are, in reality, more likely attributable to the progestins. Estrogen causes weight gain, bloating, headaches, irritability, depression, tender breasts, fatigue, thinning of scalp hair, foggy thinking, decreased libido, and most life-threatening, an increased risk of strokes. Adding the progestins to the mix gives some benefits, but once again you get bloating, headaches, weight gain, breast tenderness and depression. You also get migraines, asthma, breakthrough bleeding, liver damage, decreased glucose tolerance, excess hair growth, and an increased risk of stroke. Furthermore, *every* risk factor for breast cancer is directly or indirectly related to estrogen.

As I mentioned in the earlier chapters on hormones, there is vast difference between the synthetic progestins and natural progesterone as made by the ovary. The progestins have a long list of negative side effects, including possible miscarriage and fetal malformation, while progesterone is essential for a successful pregnancy. This alone should be a major clue to physicians and their patients that these two drugs are very, very different.

Sadly, very few studies have been done with progesterone, as it is a natural substance and therefore not patentable and profitable. Those that have been done show no side effects aside from some sleepiness at very high doses, and many benefits, especially for menopausal women.

DOES ESTROGEN REALLY PROTECT AGAINST HEART DISEASE?

That estrogen protects against heart disease has become an accepted "fact" in mainstream medicine, but in reality there is little evidence to support this claim. We do know that estrogen can improve lipid profiles (raise HDL cholesterol and lower LDL cholesterol) but it's a big leap to say that therefore it must also protect against heart disease. Doctors do not (or should not) prescribe estrogen to women who are obese, diabetic, have kidney or liver disease, are at a risk for cancer or stroke, or smoke cigarettes. Therefore, the women who took estrogen in the largest study purporting to show that estrogen reduces heart disease were, by elimination, a healthier group to begin with, and less likely to have heart disease with or without the hormone replacement therapy. (Other studies also show that women who use hormone replacement therapy are more likely to be better educated and healthier.)

Furthermore, the women who took estrogen had a much higher risk of stroke, even though they were a healthier group. To the best of my knowledge, there are no other studies showing that estrogen or hormone replacement therapy of any kind truly reduces the risk of heart disease. Somehow the fact that estrogen can increase the risk of stroke never makes it into the mainstream media.

THE REAL MENOPAUSE SOLUTIONS

All of the maladies for which doctors are prescribing estrogen can be prevented and reversed with diet and lifestyle changes and, when necessary, with some natural progesterone cream (not the synthetic progestins), which has no side effects and nearly always gives all of the benefits attributed to estrogen.

It is very well known now that heart disease is one of the most preventable of all chronic diseases with diet and lifestyle changes. Why should a woman increase her risk of breast cancer by 46 percent, her risk of stroke by up to 75 percent and suffer from all the estrogen and progestin side effects, when she can accomplish the same thing naturally and increase her quality of life in every way?

Women who keep their weight within reasonable limits, who keep their fat intake low and their vegetable intake high, and who get some regular exercise, rarely suffer from distressing menopause symptoms. Those who add soy products such as soy milk and tofu to their daily diet are even less likely to complain about menopause symptoms. High soy consumption and low fat consumption are almost certainly the primary reasons that hot flashes and breast cancer are virtually unknown in Japan.

NATURAL REMEDIES FOR A HEALTHY MENOPAUSE

Your best bet for preventing and relieving menopause symptoms such as hot flashes and vaginal dryness is plenty of exercise, clean water and a nutrition-rich, low-fat diet emphasizing vegetables and soy products.

Menopause symptoms are virtually nonexistent in Japan where fat consumption is low and soy consumption is high.

Any woman with menopause symptoms such as hot flashes, night sweats, vaginal dryness, hair loss, dry skin, and decreased libido not relieved by the above lifestyle guidelines plus the vitamins below, should try natural progesterone cream. Any woman at risk for heart disease or osteoporosis should also be using natural progesterone cream. Recent research indicates that natural progesterone may also be protective against breast cancer.

A menopausal woman can use progesterone cream, as directed, three weeks out of the month, with a week off to resensitize cell receptor sites.

According to Dr. John Lee, a very small percentage of women may need a small amount of natural estrogen cream applied topically to relieve the symptoms of vaginal dryness and hot flashes. Only a small amount is needed, and after six months to a year, it can be *gradually* discontinued.

The herbs for menopausal symptoms are the same as those listed in the premenopause syndrome chapter.

VITAMINS FOR MENOPAUSAL SYMPTOMS

Vitamins for women with menopause symptoms should include:

- Vitamin B6, 100–300 mg daily
- Beta-carotene, 15,000 to 40,000 daily in divided doses
- Choline, 500 mg
- Inositol, 500 mg
- Vitamin C, 1,000 mg
- Vitamin E, 400 IU
- Magnesium, 300 mg

CHAPTER 8

Natural Remedies for Osteoporosis

Although cardiovascular disease is the leading cause of death among American women, osteoporosis is the disease they are most likely to develop as they age. Four out of ten white women in the U.S. will fracture a hip, spine, or forearm due to osteoporosis. As many as five out of ten will develop small fractures in their spine, causing great pain and a shrinking in height. This amounts to 15 to 20 million people affected by a crippling and painful disease that is almost entirely preventable and reversible.

Osteoporosis is a gradual decrease in bone mass and density that can begin as early as the teen years. Bone mass should be at its peak in our late twenties or early thirties, but thanks to a poor diet and lack of exercise, many women are already losing bone in their twenties. Bone loss occurs more rapidly in women than in men, especially right around the time of menopause, when an abrupt drop in estrogen and progesterone accelerates bone loss.

When you think of your bones you may imagine a dead skeleton, but your bones are living tissue, just like the rest of your body, and they need a good supply of nutrients and regular exercise. New bone is constantly being made, while old bone is being reabsorbed and excreted by the body. Our larger long bones, such as our arm bones and leg bones, are very dense, and they are completely replaced about every 10 to 12 years. Our less dense bones, such as our spine and the ends of our long bones, turn over every 2 to 3 years. Thus, as you can see, we always have the opportunity to be creating better bone for ourselves.

We all hear about how having enough calcium in the diet and taking estrogen can help prevent osteoporosis, but there is a much bigger nutritional and lifestyle picture to look at when we are talking about preventing this bone-robbing disease. You'll be happy to know that for the vast majority of women, there is no need to take estrogen to prevent osteoporosis.

The most important element of bones is minerals. Without minerals we don't have bones. The most important bone minerals are calcium, magnesium, potassium, phosphorus and fluoride. Equally important is the balance between the minerals. Too much phosphorus or fluoride will create poor bone structure. (Nearly all of us already ingest too much fluoride.) Without enough magnesium, the calcium can't be absorbed onto the bone. Vitamins are also involved. For example, vitamin B6 works with magnesium to get calcium onto your bones.

Some of the things that cause you to lose bone are coffee, alcohol, cigarette smoking, aluminum, diuretics, fluoride, and high-dose synthetic cortisones such as Prednisone.

The hormones testosterone, estrogen and progesterone are also actively involved in the making and unmaking of bone. Testosterone and progesterone build bone, while estrogen appears to indirectly slow bone loss.

THE DYNAMICS OF OSTEOPOROSIS

In osteoporosis, the old bone is being reabsorbed faster than new bone is being made, causing the bones to lose density and become thinner and more porous. The integrity and strength of our bones is related to bone mass and density. The bones of a woman with osteoporosis gradually become thinner and more fragile.

A progressive loss of bone mass may continue until the skeleton is no longer strong enough to support itself. When that happens, bones can spontaneously fracture. As bones become more fragile, falls or bumps that would not have hurt us before, can cause a fracture. Bone loss seems to be most severe in the spine, wrists and hips. Unfortunately there are usually no signs or symptoms of osteoporosis until a fracture occurs.

Early Signs of Osteoporosis

Sudden insomnia and restlessness
Nightly leg and foot cramps
Persistent low back pain
Gum disease, loose teeth
Gradual loss of height

Your Risk of Osteoporosis is Higher if You:

Are a woman
Have a family history of osteoporosis
Are white
Are thin
Are short
Went into menopause early
Have a low calcium intake
Don't exercise
Smoke cigarettes
Drink more than two alcohol drinks daily
Are on chronic steroid therapy (e.g. Prednisone)
Are on chronic anticonvulsant therapy
Are taking drugs which can cause dizziness
Are hyperthyroid
Eat too much animal protein

Use antacids regularly
Drink more than two cups of coffee daily

HOW AWARE OF OSTEOPOROSIS ARE YOU?

A Gallup poll sponsored by the National Osteoporosis Foundation found that:

- 75 percent of women believed they were familiar with osteoporosis, but
- 80 percent were not aware that it was responsible for disabling fractures,
- 90 percent were surprised to learn that osteoporosis frequently causes death, and
- 60 percent could not identify the risk factors of osteoporosis.

SHOULD YOU TAKE HORMONE REPLACEMENT THERAPY TO PREVENT OSTEOPOROSIS?

There is a misperception that osteoporosis begins at menopause. According to Dr. John Lee, in reality, bone mass begins declining in most women in their mid-thirties, accelerates for 3 to 5 years around the time of menopause, and then continues to decline at the rate of about 1–1.5 percent per year.

Because bone loss accelerates at menopause, and because estrogen levels decline at menopause, conventional medicine has adopted the belief that osteoporosis is an estrogen deficiency disease that can be cured with estrogen replacement therapy. This is only partly true. Once again, thanks to the courageous and pioneering work of Dr. John Lee, we have found that the missing piece of this puzzle is diet and lifestyle, plus the bone-building hormone progesterone, which drops much more precipitously at menopause than estrogen does. (When I refer to progesterone, I mean the natural hormone, not the synthetic progestins.)

There is no question that estrogen can slow bone loss around the time of menopause, but the scientific evidence is very clear that after 5–6 years, bone loss continues at the same rate, with or without estrogen. A very large study published in the *New England Journal of Medicine* in 1995, studying risk factors for hip fractures in white women, which followed over 9500 women for eight years, found no benefit in estrogen supplementation in women over the age of 65. As Dr. Lee has pointed out, if estrogen was the only known treatment for osteoporosis, it might be worth taking it to get the small saving in bone density, despite all the risks and side effects. But since it's clear that progesterone, combined with proper diet and exercise, steadily increases bone density regardless of age, there are *very* few women who should ever need to take estrogen for osteoporosis.

PROGESTERONE AND OSTEOPOROSIS

Dr. Lee has suggested that the most important factor in osteoporosis is a lack of progesterone, which causes a decrease in new bone formation. He and others have extensive clinical experience showing that using a natural progesterone cream will actively increase bone mass and density and can *reverse* osteoporosis. After treating hundreds of patients with osteoporosis over a period of 15 years, Dr. Lee found that those women with the lowest bone densities experienced the greatest relative improvement, and those who had good bone density to begin with, maintained their strong bones.

Postmenopausal women using a transdermal (on the skin) progesterone cream or oil should use the equivalent of 20–40 mg daily for three weeks out of the month, with a week off each month to maintain the sensitivity of the progesterone receptors.

DIETARY GUIDELINES FOR AN OSTEOPOROSIS-FREE OLD AGE

Getting adequate calcium is only a small part of the dietary prevention picture for osteoporosis. Slowing the excretion of calcium is much more important than getting enough calcium in the diet. The primary factors in calcium depletion in American women are high protein diets, soda pop and antacids. Advertising that antacids can be taken for their calcium is false advertising, because antacids actually deplete calcium, so at best you're replacing what you lose when you take the antacid!

It is important for women to make sure they're getting adequate calcium. Some good food sources of calcium are snow peas, broccoli, leafy green vegetables such as spinach, kale, beet and turnip greens; almonds, figs, beans (soybeans are the best), nonfat milk, yogurt and cottage cheese. I don't want you to depend on milk to get your calcium. This is because milk has a poor calcium-to-magnesium ratio. Your body needs a certain amount of magnesium in order to get the calcium into your bones—without magnesium, calcium can't build strong bones.

In fact, magnesium deficiency may be more common in women with osteoporosis than calcium deficiency. Although many fruits and vegetables have some magnesium in them, especially good sources of magnesium are whole grains, wheat bran, leafy green vegetables, nuts (almonds are a very rich source of magnesium and calcium), beans, bananas and apricots.

Trace minerals are also important in helping your body absorb calcium. Eating plenty of green leafy vegetables gives you calcium along with these helpful trace minerals. Boron and manganese are especially important. Foods that contain boron include apples, legumes, almonds, pears and green, leafy vegetables. Foods that include manganese include ginger, buckwheat and oats.

USE 'EM OR LOSE 'EM

Lack of exercise is one of the primary causes of osteoporosis. Using your bones keeps them strong and healthy. Weight-bearing exercise is the only thing besides progesterone found to actually *increase* bone density in older women. By weight-bearing I mean exercise that uses your bones. Brisk walking counts as weight-bearing exercise, but add some hand-held weights and it's even better. Pushing a vacuum cleaner or lawn mower, gardening, dancing, and aerobic exercise also qualify.

Your exercise plan should include a minimum of 20 minutes of weight-bearing exercise three to four times a week. An hour is even better. In contrast to women who exercise, those who don't continue to lose bone, regardless of what else they are doing. Studies of elderly people who fall and break a bone show that these people had poor flexibility, poor leg strength, instability when first standing, and difficulty getting up and down in a chair.

Exercise can help increase flexibility, strength, and coordination. A weight lifting program of just half an hour three to four times a week can significantly improve bone density. You don't need to go to the gym to do a weight lifting program. You can lift a can of peas or a small carton of milk.

Women with advanced osteoporosis should work with a physical therapist to create a safe, effective program to reduce the risk of fracture. The Asian movement exercises such as yoga, tai chi and chi gong can also be excellent for improving strength, flexibility and coordination.

SUNSHINE IS THE BEST MEDICINE

Vitamin D is another important ingredient in the recipe for strong bones because it stimulates the absorption of calcium. A deficiency of vitamin D can cause calcium loss. The best way to get vitamin D is from direct sunlight on the skin. Sunlight stimulates a chain of events in the skin leading to the production of vitamin D in the liver and kidneys. (This is why liver and kidney disease can produce a vitamin D deficiency.) Going outside for just a few minutes a day can give us all the vitamin D we need, and yet many people don't even do that. They go from their home, to their car, to their office, and back home, without spending more than a few seconds outdoors. Many elderly people are unable to get outside without assistance, but this should be a priority for their caretakers.

THE COLLAGEN VITAMINS AND MINERALS

Collagen is the tissue that makes up your bone. To build collagen you need vitamin A (or beta-carotene), zinc and vitamin C. Vitamin C is especially important, as it is the primary ingredient in the collagen matrix. I recommend you take 1,000 to 2,000 mg daily of vitamin C, in an esterified form to prevent stomach problems.

SUPPLEMENTS FOR BONE BUILDING

Calcium, 1,200 to 1,500 mg daily with meals
Magnesium glycinate, 600-900 mg daily with meals
Folic acid, 200 mcg daily

Vitamin C, 1,000–2,000 mg twice daily
Vitamin B6, 50–100 mg daily between meals
Zinc, 15 mg daily with meals
Beta carotene, 15,000 IU daily
Trace minerals, including 1–3 mg of boron and manganese

HERBS FOR BONE BUILDING

Oatstraw *(Avena sativa)* is high in silica, which enhances calcium absorption.
Horsetail *(Equisetum arvense)* is high in silica, which enhances calcium absorption.

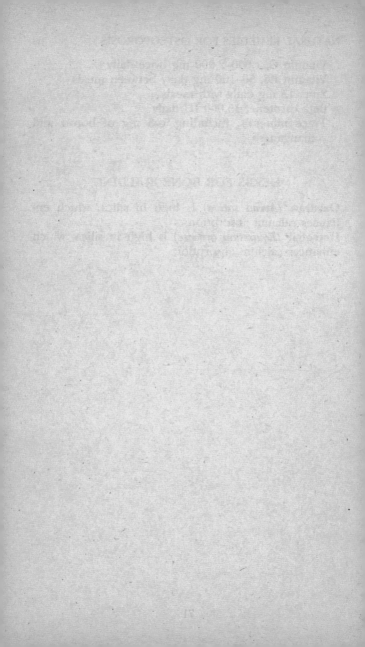

SOURCES FOR NATURAL PROGESTERONE CREAM

Kenogen, P.O. Box 5764, Eugene, OR 97405, (503) 345-9855. This is progesterone in vitamin E oil, called Progest-E Complex.

Professional & Technical Services, Inc., 621 S.W. Alder, Suite 900, Portland, Oregon 97205-3627. (503) 226-1010, (800) 888-6814. They sell Pro-Gest, the best known of the progesterone creams.

RESOURCES AND RECOMMENDED READING

The Biologic Role of Dehydroepiandrosterone, editors M. Kalimi and W. Regelson, publisher Walter de Gruyter, 1990.

Breast Cancer: What You Should Know (But May Not Be Told) About Prevention, Diagnosis, and Treatment by Steve Austin, N.D., and Cathy Hitchcock, M.S.W., Prima Publishing, P.O. Box 1260BK, Rocklin, CA 95677, 1992.

Cowan LD, Gordis L, Tonascia JA, Jones GS. Breast cancer incidence in women with a history of progesterone deficiency. Am J Epidemiology 1981; 114:209-217.

Earl Mindell's Soy Miracle by Earl Mindell, R.Ph., Ph.D., Simon & Schuster, New York, 1995.

"Effects of estrogen or estrogen/progestin regimens on heart disease risk factors in postmenopausal women," The postmenopausal estrogen/progestins interventions (PEPI) trial, January 18, 1995, JAMA.

Ellison P.T., Panter-Brick C., Lipson S.F. and O'Rourke M.T., "The ecological context of human ovarian function," Human Reproduction, 1993; 8:2248-58.)

Encyclopedia of Natural Medicine by Michael Murray, N.D. and Joseph Pizzorno, N.D., Prima Publishing, 1991.

Felson DT, Zhang Y, Hannan MT, Kiel DP, Wilson PWF, Anderson JJ, "The effect of postmenopausal estrogen therapy on bone density in elderly women," N Engl J Med 1993; 329:1141-1146.

Hammond CB, Jelvsek FR, Lee KL, Creasman WT, Parker RT, "Effects of long-term estrogen replacement therapy, I. Metabolic effects," Am J Ob-Gyn 1979; 133:525-536.

Hedlund LR, Gallagher JC, "Increased incidence of hip fracture in osteoporotic women treated with sodium fluoride," J Bone & Miner Res 1989; 4:223-225.

Hileman B. "Reproductive Estrogens Linked to Reproductive Abnormalities, Cancer," Chemical and Engineering News, January 31, 1994, p. 19-23.

Hormone Replacement Therapy: Yes or No? by Betty Kamen, Nutrition Encounter, Inc., publisher, P.O. Box 5847, Novato, CA 94948, 1993.

The Hysterectomy Hoax by Stanley West, M.D., Doubleday, New York, 1994.

Kleerekoper ME, Peterson E, Phillips E, Nelson D, et al. "Continuous sodium fluoride therapy does not reduce vertebral fracture rate in postmenopausal osteoporosis [abstract]," J Bone Miner Res 1989; Res. 4 (Suppl. 1):S376.

The Mindell Letter, Philips Publishing Inc., 7811 Montrose Rd., Potomac, MD 20854, or call (800) 787-3003.

Natural Pest Control, by Andrew Lopez, The Invisible Gardner of Malibu, 29161 Heathercliff Road, Ste. 216-408, Malibu, CA 90265, (800) 354-9296.

Preventing and Reversing Osteoporosis, Alan R. Gaby MD, Prima Publishing, 1993.

Prior JC, Progesterone as a bone-trophic hormone. Endocr Rev 1990; 11:386-398.

Prior JC, Postmenopausal estrogen therapy and cardiovascular disease (Letter). N Engl J Med 1991; 326:705-706.

Prior JC, Vigna YM, Alojado N, "Progesterone and

the prevention of osteoporosis," Canadian J of Ob/ Gyn & Women Health Care 1991; 3:178-184.

Prior JC, "Progesterone as a bone-trophic hormone," Endocrine Reviews 1990; 11:386-398.) Horm Res 1992;37:132-6.

Raloff, J., "Ecocancers, " Science News, Vol. 144, July 3, 1993, p. 10-13.

Raloff, J., "The Gender Benders," Science News, Vol. 145, January 8, 1994, p. 24-27.

Raloff, J., "That Feminine Touch," Science News, Vol. 145, January 22, 1994, p. 56-59.

Sherman BM, West JH, Korenmam SG. The menopausal transition: analysis of LH, FSH, estradiol and progesterone concentrations during menstrual cycles of older women. J Clin Endocrinol Metab 1976;42:629-636.

Stampfer M.J., Coditz G.A., Willet W.C., et al, "Postmenopausal estrogen therapy and cardiovascular disease—ten-year follow-up from the Nurses' Health Study," N Engl J Med, 1991;325:756-762.

What Your Doctor May Not Tell You About Menopause: The Breakthrough Book on Natural Progesterone, John R. Lee, M.D. with Virginia Hopkins, Warner Books, New York, 1996.

Women's Bodies, Women's Wisdom, Christiane Northrup MD, Bantam Books, New York, 1994.

GLOSSARY

adrenal glands The glands, located above each kidney, that manufacture **adrenalin(e)**, **noradrenalin(e)**, and **steroids**.

adrenalin(e) A hormone secreted by the **adrenal glands** into the bloodstream in response to physical or mental stress, such as fear or injury; works with **noradrenalin(e)** to regulate blood pressure and heart rate.

aldosterone A hormone secreted by the **adrenal glands** which regulates the salt and water balance in the body; one of the **steroids**.

alkaline Containing an acid-neutralizing substance (being alkaline, sodium bicarbonate is used for excess acidity in foods).

amino acids The organic compounds from which proteins are constructed; 22 amino acids have been identified as necessary to the human body; nine are known as essential—histidine, isoleucine, leucine, lysine, total S-containing amino acids, total aromatic amino acids, threonine, tryptophan, and valine—and must be obtained from food.

amenorrhea Absence or suppression of menstruation.

androgen Any of the group of hormones which stimulates male characteristics.

antihistamine A drug used to reduce effects associated with histamine production in allergies and colds.

antioxidant A substance that can protect another substance from **oxidation**; added to foods to keep oxygen from changing the food's color.

arteriosclerosis A disease of the arteries characterized by hardening, thickening and loss of elasticity of the arterial walls; results in impaired blood circulation.

beta-carotene A plant pigment which can be converted into two forms of **vitamin** A.

bioflavonoids A group of compounds needed to maintain healthy blood vessel walls; found chiefly as coloring matter in flowers and fruits, particularly yellow ones; known as vitamin P complex.

biotin A colorless, crystalline B complex **vitamin**; essential for the activity of many **enzyme** systems; helps produce **fatty acids**; found in large quantities in liver, egg yolk, milk, and yeast.

capillary A minute blood vessel, one of many that connect the arteries and veins and deliver oxygen to tissues.

carcinogen A cancer-causing substance.

cardiovascular Relating to the heart and blood vessels.

carotene An orange-yellow pigment occurring in many plants and capable of being converted into **vitamin** A in the body.

cholesterol A white, crystalline substance, made up of various fats; naturally produced in vertebrate animals and humans; important as a precursor to steroid hormones and as a constituent of cell membranes.

chronic Of long duration, continuing, constant.

CNS Central nervous system.

coenzyme A substance that combines with other substances to form a complete **enzyme**; nonprotein and usually a B **vitamin**.

collagen The primary **organic** constituent of bone, cartilage and connective tissue (becomes gelatin through boiling).

complex carbohydrate Fibrous molecules of starch or sugar which slowly release sugar into the bloodstream.

corticosteroids See **steroids.**

demineralization The loss of minerals or salts from bone and tissue.

diuretic Tending to increase the flow of urine from the body.

endocrine Producing secretions passed directly to the **lymph** or blood instead of into a duct; to do with the endocrine glands or the **hormones** they produce.

endorphins Natural opiates produced in the brain; pain suppressants.

enzyme A **protein** substance found in living cells that brings about chemical changes; necessary for digestion of food; compounds with names ending in -ase.

epinephrine See **adrenalin(e)**

fatty acids Acids produced by the breakdown of fats; essential fatty acids cannot be produced by the body and must be included in the diet.

free radicals Highly reactive chemical fragments that can beneficially act as chemical messengers, but in excess produce an irritation of artery walls and start the arteriosclerotic process if antioxidants are not present.

fructose A natural sugar occurring in fruits and honey; called fruit sugar; often used as a preservative for foodstuffs and an intravenous nutrient.

gland An organ in the body where certain substances in the blood are separated and converted into secretions for use in the body (such as hormones) or to be discharged from the body (such as sweat); nonsecreting structures similar to glands, like **lymph** nodes, are also known as glands.

glucose Blood sugar; a product of the body's assimilation of carbohydrates and a major source of energy.

HDL High-density lipoprotein; HDL is sometimes called "good" **cholesterol** because it is the body's major carrier of cholesterol to the liver for excretion in the bile.

hesperidin Part of the **vitamin** C complex.

hormone A substance formed in **endocrine** organs and transported by body fluids to activate other specifically receptive organs, cells or tissues.

hyperglycemia A condition caused by high blood sugar.

hypoglycemia A condition caused by abnormally low blood sugar.

insulin A **hormone**, secreted by the pancreas, that helps regulate the **metabolism** of sugar in the body.

IU International Units

lactose One of the sugars found in milk.

LDL Low-density lipoprotein; sometimes referred to as "bad" **cholesterol**, LDLs easily become **oxidized** and carry cholesterol through the bloodstream; studies show high levels can increase risk of coronary artery disease (CAD).

lecithin Any of a group of fats rich in phosphorus; essential for transforming fats in the body; rich sources include egg yolk, soybeans and corn.

linoleic acid One of the polyunsaturated fats; an essential **fatty acid**; a constituent of **lecithin**; known as **vitamin** F; indispensable for life, and must be obtained from foods.

lipid A fat or fatty substance.

lipotropic Preventing abnormal or excessive accumulation of fat; lipotropin is a **hormone** which stimulates the conversion of stored fat to usable, liquid form.

lymph The almost clear fluid flowing through the lymphatic vessels; lymph nourishes tissue cells and returns waste matter to the bloodstream.

lymph nodes, spleen, thymus, and tonsils; lymphocytes make up between 22 and 28 percent of adult human white blood cells; primarily responsible for **antibody** production, lymphocytes include **B cells** and **T cells**.

metabolism The processes of physical and chemical change where food is synthesized into living matter until it is broken down into simpler substances or waste matter; energy is produced by these processes.

neurotransmitter A chemical substance which transmits or changes nerve impulses.

noradrenalin(e) A hormone produced in the **adrenal glands** that increases blood pressure by blood vessel narrowing without affecting the heart's output; works with **epinephrine**.

norepinephrine See **noradrenalin(e)**.

organic Describes any chemical containing carbon; or any food or supplement made with animal or vegetable fertilizers; or produced without synthetic fertilizers or pesticides and free from chemical injections or additives.

oxalates **Organic** chemicals found in certain foods, especially spinach, which can combine with calcium to form calcium oxalate, an insoluble chemical the body cannot use.

oxidation The way in which certain types of altered

oxygen molecules cause biochemical reactions; examples are browning of apples and rancidity in oil.

peroxides   Free radicals formed as by-products when oxygen reacts with molecules of fat.

phytoestrogen Any of a number of compounds found in plants which occupy estrogen receptors and may help protect the body from the negative effects of excess estrogen.

placebo A substance which produces no pharmacological activity; one which is used instead of and alongside an active substance for comparison.

polysaccharides A molecule made up of many sugar molecules joined together.

polyunsaturated fats Highly nonsaturated fats from vegetable sources; can dissolve or absorb other substances.

prostaglandins Hormone-like substances that aid in regulation of the immune system.

protein A complex substance containing nitrogen which is essential to plant and animal cells; ingested proteins are changed to **amino acids** in the body.

PUFA Polyunsaturated **fatty acid**.

saturated fatty acids Usually solid at room temperature; higher proportions found in foods from animal sources.

serotonin A **neurotransmitter** considered essential for sleep and concentration.

simple carbohydrate Simple sugar molecules, such as **glucose**, which are rapidly absorbed by the bloodstream.

steroids   Hormones produced by the **adrenal glands** that influence or control key functions of the body;

formed from **cholesterol**; three major types influencing skin, muscle, fat, and **metabolism** of **glucose**, sexual functions and characteristics, and processing of minerals; used as drugs such as cortisone to suppress the immune system, reduce inflammation and to treat allergies.

synergistic The way two or more substances produce an effect that neither alone could accomplish.

synthetic Produced artificially; not found in nature.

systemic Capable of spreading through the entire body.

tocopherols The group of compounds (alpha, beta, delta, epsilon, eta, gamma and zeta) that make **vitamin** E; obtained through vacuum distillation of edible vegetable oils.

toxicity The quality or condition of being poisonous, harmful, or destructive.

toxin An **organic** poison produced in living or dead organisms.

triglycerides Fatty substances in the blood.

unsaturated fatty acids Most often liquid at room temperature; primarily found in vegetable fats.

virus Any of a large group of minute organisms that can only reproduce in the cells of plants and animals.

vitamin Any of about fifteen natural compounds essential in small amounts as catalysts for processes in the body; most cannot be made by the body and must come from diet.

yeast Single-celled fungus that can cause infections in the body.

INDEX

Dr. Earl Mindell's

What You Should Know About . . .
series
in print or forthcoming

Beautiful Hair, Skin and Nails

Better Nutrition for Athletes

Fiber and Digestion

Herbs for Your Health

Homeopathic Remedies

Natural Health for Men

Natural Health for Women

Nutrition for Active Lifestyles

The Super Antioxidant Miracle

Trace Minerals

22 Ways to a Healthier Heart